Amish Herbal Remedies & Apothecary

A Beginner's Quick Start Guide to Natural Healing with a 7-Step Action Plan and Sample Traditional Recipes

mf

copyright © 2025 Mary Golanna

All rights reserved No part of this book may be reproduced, or stored in a retrieval system, or transmitted in any form or by any means, electronic, mechanical, photocopying, recording, or otherwise, without express written permission of the publisher.

Disclaimer

By reading this disclaimer, you are accepting the terms of the disclaimer in full. If you disagree with this disclaimer, please do not read the guide.

All of the content within this guide is provided for informational and educational purposes only, and should not be accepted as independent medical or other professional advice. The author is not a doctor, physician, nurse, mental health provider, or registered nutritionist/dietician. Therefore, using and reading this guide does not establish any form of a physician-patient relationship.

Always consult with a physician or another qualified health provider with any issues or questions you might have regarding any sort of medical condition. Do not ever disregard any qualified professional medical advice or delay seeking that advice because of anything you have read in this guide. The information in this guide is not intended to be any sort of medical advice and should not be used in lieu of any medical advice by a licensed and qualified medical professional.

The information in this guide has been compiled from a variety of known sources. However, the author cannot attest to or guarantee the accuracy of each source and thus should not be held liable for any errors or omissions.

You acknowledge that the publisher of this guide will not be held liable for any loss or damage of any kind incurred as a result of this guide or the reliance on any information provided within this guide. You acknowledge and agree that you assume all risk and responsibility for any action you undertake in response to the information in this guide.

Using this guide does not guarantee any particular result (e.g., weight loss or a cure). By reading this guide, you acknowledge that there are no guarantees to any specific outcome or results you can expect.

All product names, diet plans, or names used in this guide are for identification purposes only and are the property of their respective owners. The use of these names does not imply endorsement. All other trademarks cited herein are the property of their respective owners.

Where applicable, this guide is not intended to be a substitute for the original work of this diet plan and is, at most, a supplement to the original work for this diet plan and never a direct substitute. This guide is a personal expression of the facts of that diet plan.

Where applicable, persons shown in the cover images are stock photography models and the publisher has obtained the rights to use the images through license agreements with third-party stock image companies.

Table of Contents

Introduction 7
Understanding the Amish Approach to Natural Healing 9
    The Role of Herbs in Amish Culture 10
    Benefits of Incorporating Herbal Remedies into Modern Life 11
Essential Amish Herbs and Their Uses 13
    Echinacea (Echinacea purpurea) 13
    Peppermint (Mentha × piperita) 14
    Chamomile (Matricaria chamomilla) 15
    Lavender (Lavandula angustifolia) 16
        Applications 16
    Calendula (Calendula officinalis) 16
    Yarrow (Achillea millefolium) 17
    Elderberry (Sambucus nigra) 18
    Cultivation and Harvesting Techniques 18
Preparing Herbal Remedies at Home 21
    Methods for Creating Teas, Tinctures, Salves, and Poultices 21
    Proper Dosage and Storage Practices 26
    Tools and Equipment Needed 27
7-Step Action Plan to Incorporate Amish Herbal Remedies 29
    Step 1: Assess Your Personal Health Needs 29
    Step 2: Selecting Appropriate Herbs 33
    Step 3: Sourcing Quality Ingredients 37
    Step 4: Preparing Remedies 41
    Step 5: Integrating Remedies into Daily Routines 45
    Step 6: Monitoring and Documenting Effects 50
    Step 7: Adjusting and Customizing Your Approach 55
Sample Recipes for Common Ailments 61
    Herbal Tea Blends for Colds and Flu 62
    Soothing Salves for Aches and Pains 67

Natural Solutions for Digestive Issues	72
Safety Considerations and Best Practices for Using Amish Herbal Remedies	**77**
Understanding Potential Side Effects	77
Consulting with Healthcare Professionals	79
Responsible Use of Herbal Remedies	81
Integrating Amish Remedies with Modern Wellness	**84**
Combining Traditional Wisdom with Modern Practices	84
Creating a Balanced and Holistic Lifestyle	86
Resources and Further Reading	**91**
Recommended Books and Publications	91
Online Communities and Workshops	92
Connecting with Practitioners	93
Conclusion	**97**
FAQs	**100**
References and Helpful Links	**103**

Introduction

Amish herbal remedies offer a chance to reconnect with nature while exploring time-tested approaches to health and wellness. Rooted in traditions that emphasize simplicity, self-sufficiency, and a deep bond with the earth, these remedies provide practical ways to support the body and mind using natural ingredients.

The Amish approach to healing reflects a philosophy of prevention, balance, and treating the root cause of ailments, offering valuable insights that align with today's growing interest in holistic health.

From medicinal gardens to generational knowledge passed down through families, the Amish prioritize mindfulness in crafting and using their remedies. Herbs are more than just tools for wellness; they symbolize a commitment to living harmoniously with nature and fostering a sustainable lifestyle. Their methods are straightforward, requiring minimal equipment, and rely heavily on the quality of ingredients, making them accessible to anyone interested in natural health practices.

In this guide, we will talk about the following:

- Understanding the Amish Approach to Natural Healing
- Essential Amish Herbs and Their Uses
- Preparing Herbal Remedies at Home
- 7-Step Action Plan to Incorporate Amish Herbal Remedies
- Sample Recipes for Common Ailments
- Safety Considerations and Best Practices for Using Amish Herbal Remedies
- Integrating Amish Remedies with Modern Wellness

Keep reading to discover how Amish herbal remedies can empower you to take control of your health and well-being. By the end of this guide, you will have a better understanding of the Amish approach to natural healing and how it can benefit your life.

Understanding the Amish Approach to Natural Healing

The Amish are known for their simple, traditional way of life, and their approach to health reflects these values. They focus on natural therapies, especially herbal remedies, as a way to maintain and restore health. Instead of relying on modern pharmaceutical drugs, they turn to the earth, believing that it provides everything needed to stay well.

Key features of the Amish healing approach include:

- *Focus on prevention*: They use wholesome diets, natural remedies, and simple living to avoid illnesses.
- *Treating the root cause*: Instead of only dealing with symptoms, they aim to solve the problem at its source.
- *Gentle treatments*: Herbal remedies are used because they are effective without being harsh on the body.
- *Simplicity and safety*: Their methods involve straightforward preparations with an emphasis on quality.

This philosophy aligns with holistic healing systems, where the priority is to balance and nurture health long-term.

The Role of Herbs in Amish Culture

Herbs play a vital role in Amish life. They are not just medicines but symbols of independence, self-sufficiency, and a connection to nature.

Importance of Herbs:

- Medicinal gardens are common in Amish homes, where families grow plants for specific health benefits.
- Generational knowledge is highly valued. Parents pass down skills related to growing, identifying, and using herbs to their children.
- Common uses include remedies for fevers, colds, digestion, stress, and wounds.

Key Values Behind Herbal Practices:

- *Self-sufficiency:* Growing and preparing their own remedies reduces reliance on store-bought products.
- *Simplicity:* Methods are straightforward and avoid unnecessary chemicals.
- *Mindfulness:* The process of tending and using herbs fosters a spiritual connection with nature and gratitude for its gifts.

Herbs are deeply woven into Amish culture, representing both practical health solutions and a philosophy of living in harmony with the earth.

Benefits of Incorporating Herbal Remedies into Modern Life

Amish wisdom about herbal remedies can easily be applied in today's world. These natural methods offer a refreshing alternative to complicated and sometimes harmful modern options.

Why Herbal Remedies Work:

- *Gentle and effective:* Many herbs help with conditions like colds, bloating, or anxiety without the side effects of synthetic drugs.
- *Focus on prevention:* Using herbs like echinacea regularly can support immunity and overall well-being.
- *Cost-effective and accessible:* Many remedies are simple to prepare and come from ingredients that can be easily grown or bought.

Additional Benefits:

- *Encourages mindfulness:* Preparing teas or salves takes time and care, helping you slow down and focus on your health.
- *Promotes balance:* Incorporating herbs can improve physical, emotional, and even spiritual well-being.

Herbs like chamomile for relaxation or peppermint for digestion are easy to start using. Even small steps, like enjoying a daily herbal tea or growing a few herbs in your garden, can make a difference.

Essential Amish Herbs and Their Uses

Herbs are at the heart of Amish healing traditions, treasured for their medicinal properties and the connection they foster with nature. The diversity of herbs used in Amish practices reflects centuries of accumulated wisdom and experimentation. This chapter explores some of the most popular herbs in greater depth, along with practical advice on how to cultivate and harvest them to get the best out of their natural healing powers.

Echinacea (Echinacea purpurea)

Medicinal Properties

Echinacea is a star in herbal medicine, especially valued for its immune-boosting properties. It stimulates the body's defense mechanisms, helping to fend off colds, respiratory infections, and other illnesses. Rich in antioxidants, echinacea also encourages better wound healing and combats inflammation.

Applications

- *Immune Support:* Brew it as a tea or take it as a tincture to strengthen immunity during flu season.
- *Wound Healing:* Use it as an infused oil to treat minor scrapes and cuts.

Cultural Significance

Echinacea, known to some Amish healers as "snakeroot," has been used not only as medicine but also as a symbol of nature's ability to restore health.

Peppermint (Mentha × piperita)

Medicinal Properties

Peppermint is one of the most versatile herbs in Amish herbalism. Its high menthol content makes it a go-to for soothing digestion, easing headaches, and relieving muscle tension. It also has mild antibacterial properties.

Applications

- *Digestive Support:* Brew a peppermint tea to relieve gas or bloating.
- *Headache Relief:* Rub diluted peppermint essential oil on the temples for tension and sinus headaches.
- *Muscle Aches:* Add peppermint to salves for cooling sore muscles.

Cultural Significance

Peppermint is often planted near Amish homes as a sign of hospitality and also serves as a companion plant in gardens due to its pest-repelling properties.

Chamomile (Matricaria chamomilla)

Medicinal Properties

Chamomile is cherished for its calming effects on both the body and mind. It helps with digestion, sleep issues, and inflammation, and its gentle nature makes it suitable for children. Chamomile is also revered for easing skin irritations.

Applications

- *Sleep Aid:* Drink a warm cup of chamomile tea before bed to encourage rest.
- *Skin Relief:* Prepare a compress to reduce skin redness, rashes, or minor burns.
- *Stress Reduction:* Create a bath soak with dried chamomile flowers.

Cultural Significance

Chamomile is seen as an herb of peace within Amish homes and is often used in calming remedies for family members of all ages.

Lavender (Lavandula angustifolia)

Medicinal Properties

Lavender is a favorite among Amish healers for its ability to relax the mind, promote sleep, and reduce anxiety. Additionally, it has antiseptic and healing properties, making it useful for skin issues and minor wounds.

Applications

- ***Calming Remedy:*** Use lavender in sachets, teas, and essential oils to ease stress and insomnia.
- ***Skincare:*** Add lavender-infused oil to lotions for soothing irritated skin.
- ***Natural Cleaner:*** Create a lavender spray to sanitize surfaces at home.

Cultural Significance

Among the Amish, lavender is often associated with cleanliness and order. Lavender bouquets may be placed in homes for their pleasant aroma and calming presence.

Calendula (Calendula officinalis)

Medicinal Properties

Also known as marigold, calendula is a must-have in the Amish herbalist's toolkit. It's prized for its anti-inflammatory, antibacterial, and antifungal properties. Calendula also promotes tissue repair, making it ideal for skin ailments.

Applications

- **Wound Care:** Use calendula salves or poultices to speed the healing of cuts and burns.
- **Digestive Health:** Make calendula tea to soothe upset stomachs.
- **Skincare:** Add calendula to bathwater for extra hydration and comfort to dry skin.

Cultural Significance

Calendula is often referred to as "sun's bride" in Amish gardens for its warm orange blooms and its sunny, cheerful presence.

Yarrow (Achillea millefolium)

Medicinal Properties

Yarrow is well-regarded for its ability to staunch bleeding, relieve fevers, and aid in faster recovery from illness. Its astringent and anti-inflammatory properties also lend themselves to treating wounds and skin irritations.

Applications

- **First Aid:** Apply fresh yarrow leaves to cuts and wounds as a field remedy.
- **Respiratory Health:** Prepare yarrow tea to help with colds or flu.
- **Skin Healing:** Use as a poultice for bruises and boils.

Cultural Significance

Yarrow is sometimes seen as a "warrior's herb" in Amish culture for its historical use in battlefield first aid.

Elderberry (Sambucus nigra)

Medicinal Properties

Elderberries are packed with antioxidants and vitamins that support immune health. They are most commonly used to prevent or shorten colds and the flu.

Applications

- *Cold Prevention:* Make elderberry syrups or gummies to be taken daily during cold seasons.
- *Fever Relief:* Drink elderberry tea to combat fevers.
- *Anti-Inflammatory:* Use elderberry tinctures to help reduce inflammation post-illness.

Cultural Significance

Elder trees have long been considered protectors of the home in Amish lore, and elderberries are treasured as one of the most potent berries in their herbal traditions.

Cultivation and Harvesting Techniques

While the Amish are known for their resourcefulness and self-sufficient farming, their methods of cultivating herbs are often grounded in basic principles that anyone can follow.

Soil Preparation

- Before planting, test the soil in your garden. Herbs typically thrive in well-draining soil with a slightly neutral to slightly alkaline pH (6.5-7.5).
- Enrich the soil with compost or aged manure to ensure the herbs have plenty of nutrients.

Planting and Seasonal Care

- Herbs such as chamomile, mint, and calendula flourish in full sun. To get the best results, find a spot that receives 6–8 hours of direct sunlight daily.
- Many herbs are best planted in early spring, but some (like elderberries) may require fall planting depending on your local climate.

Pest Management

- The Amish rely heavily on natural pest deterrents like companion planting. For example, planting basil and marigold near other herbs can deter aphids and other pests.
- Make simple herbal sprays from garlic and neem to repel insects without harmful chemicals.

Watering and Maintenance

- Most herbs prefer moderate watering. Water deeply and allow the soil to dry partially before watering

- again. Overwatering can harm plants like lavender and echinacea.
- Mulch around your plants to conserve moisture and prevent weeds.

Harvesting Tips

- Herbs are most potent just before flowering. This is when their oils and beneficial compounds are at their peak.
- Use pruning shears to cut herbs early in the morning, as this is when they are most hydrated.
- For root-based herbs like echinacea, harvest in late fall when the plant's nutrients are primarily stored in the roots.

By incorporating these planting and harvesting techniques, you'll be able to maintain a thriving herbal garden that's not only bountiful but truly reflective of the Amish tradition of stewardship and care for nature.

Preparing Herbal Remedies at Home

One of the most fulfilling aspects of exploring herbal remedies is learning to prepare them yourself. This hands-on process not only gives you control over what you consume but also connects you to the remedies and their natural origins.

From simple teas to healing salves, this chapter will guide you through the methods, tools, and practices essential for creating your own herbal remedies at home. We'll also cover proper dosing, storage, and safety tips to ensure your preparations are both effective and long-lasting.

Methods for Creating Teas, Tinctures, Salves, and Poultices

Herbal Teas

Herbal teas are the easiest and most popular way to enjoy the healing benefits of herbs. They extract the water-soluble compounds from the herb and are soothing, warming, and highly customizable.

Step-by-Step Instructions:

1. ***Choose Your Herb(s):*** Use one or a blend of herbs. Start with 1 teaspoon of dried herbs or 1 tablespoon of fresh herbs per 8 ounces of water. For example, chamomile tea can calm the mind, or peppermint tea can ease digestion.

2. ***Boil Water:*** Bring water to a boil, then pour it over your herbs in a teacup, mug, or teapot.

3. ***Steep:*** Cover the cup to trap the heat and allow the herbs to steep for 10-15 minutes for maximum potency.

4. ***Strain and Serve:*** Use a fine mesh strainer or tea infuser to remove the herbs. Sweeten with honey if desired and enjoy.

Tips for Beginners:

- Experiment with herbal combinations to balance flavors and maximize health benefits (e.g., ginger and mint for nausea).
- For a stronger infusion, use 2 teaspoons of herbs and steep for up to 20 minutes.

Tinctures

Tinctures are concentrated herbal extracts made by soaking herbs in alcohol or vinegar. They are versatile, long-lasting, and easy to administer in small doses.

Step-by-Step Instructions:

1. *Gather Ingredients:* You'll need dried or fresh herbs, alcohol (vodka or brandy with at least 80-proof), a mason jar, and a dropper bottle.
2. *Prepare the Jar:* Fill a clean glass jar halfway with your chosen herb.
3. *Add Alcohol:* Pour alcohol over the herbs until they are completely submerged, leaving about an inch of space at the top.
4. *Seal and Shake:* Secure the lid tightly and shake the jar. Label it with the date and contents.
5. *Steep:* Store the jar in a cool, dark place for 4-6 weeks. Shake daily to ensure the herb is evenly absorbed.
6. *Strain:* After steeping, strain the tincture through cheesecloth into a clean jar or bowl. Transfer to dropper bottles for easy use.

Tips for Beginners:

- Use vinegar or glycerin as a substitute for alcohol when making tinctures for children.

- Typical tincture dosage is 1-2 droppers full (20-40 drops) diluted in water or juice. Always start with a small dose to gauge your body's reaction.

Salves

Salves are soothing, oil-based remedies ideal for topical applications like healing wounds, treating dry skin, or relieving sore muscles.

Step-by-Step Instructions:

1. *Make Herbal Oil:* Infuse herbs like calendula or comfrey in oil first. Fill a jar halfway with dried herbs and top with carrier oil (e.g., olive or coconut oil). Seal and leave in a sunny spot for 2-4 weeks, shaking occasionally.
2. *Melt the Beeswax:* Heat your infused oil in a double boiler, then add grated beeswax. The general ratio is 1 ounce of beeswax for every cup of oil. Stir until melted and combined.
3. *Add Essential Oils (Optional):* To enhance skin-healing properties, add 10-15 drops of essential oils like lavender.
4. *Pour and Set:* Carefully pour the liquid salve into clean tins or jars. Allow it to cool and harden before sealing.

Tips for Beginners:

- Test your salve for consistency before pouring by placing a small amount on a cold plate. If too soft, add more beeswax; if too hard, add more oil.
- Keep salves in a cool, dark spot to extend their shelf life.

Poultices

Poultices are topical applications of crushed or mashed herbs designed to draw out toxins, reduce inflammation, or alleviate pain directly at the site of injury or discomfort.

Step-by-Step Instructions:

1. *Prepare Herbs:* Use fresh or dried herbs (e.g., yarrow for wounds or chamomile for swelling). For dried herbs, rehydrate by soaking them in warm water.
2. *Mash or Crush:* Crush the herbs into a thick paste using a mortar and pestle or blender. You can mix in a small amount of water, honey, or oil to make it more cohesive.
3. *Apply to Cloth:* Place the herbal paste onto a clean gauze, cloth, or muslin. Fold the material to encase the herbs.
4. *Apply to Skin:* Place the poultice directly onto the affected area and secure it with a bandage. Leave it on for 30 minutes to 2 hours, depending on the condition.

Tips for Beginners:

- Warm poultices can soothe muscle pain, while cold poultices can reduce swelling.
- Change the poultice regularly if treating long-term conditions like bruising or infections.

Proper Dosage and Storage Practices

Dosage Guidelines

- *Start Small:* Introduce remedies gradually, starting with the lowest effective dose, and increase only as needed.
- *Consider Age and Sensitivity:* Children and sensitive individuals require milder preparations and smaller doses.
- *Consult a Healthcare Provider:* If in doubt, especially when managing chronic illnesses or during pregnancy, seek professional guidance.

Storage Best Practices

- *Teas:* Consume herbal teas fresh. If storing, refrigerate and consume within 24-48 hours.
- *Tinctures:* Store tinctures in glass dropper bottles in a cool, dark place. Properly made tinctures can last for up to 5 years.
- *Salves:* Store in airtight containers in a cool, dry location. Most salves maintain their efficacy for 1 year.

- ***Poultices:*** Poultices are disposable and should not be reused after a single application.

Tools and Equipment Needed

Having the right tools makes herbal preparation much easier and more enjoyable. Here's a beginner-friendly checklist:

1. ***Glass Jars:*** Useful for steeping tinctures, infused oils, or teas without leaching chemicals into your remedies.
2. ***Mortar and Pestle:*** Handy for crushing and grinding herbs for teas, salves, or poultices.
3. ***Fine Mesh Strainers or Cheesecloth:*** Essential for straining tinctures, salves, and teas.
4. ***Measuring Spoons and Cups:*** For precise measurements of herbs and liquids.
5. ***Double Boiler:*** Useful for gently heating salves without burning the oil.
6. ***Reusable Tea Bags or Infusers:*** Ideal for making single servings of herbal tea.
7. ***Dropper Bottles:*** Perfect for storing tinctures and controlling dosages.
8. ***Sharp Scissors or Pruners:*** For harvesting herbs from your garden.
9. ***Labels and Markers:*** Clearly label containers with the remedy name, date, and ingredients to avoid confusion.

With these tools and methods, you'll have everything you need to begin crafting your own herbal remedies. Not only will you save money compared to store-bought alternatives, but you'll also gain confidence and joy in the process of creating personalized, natural solutions for your health.

7-Step Action Plan to Incorporate Amish Herbal Remedies

The Amish have a long history of using herbs to support health naturally. You don't have to live off the land to benefit from their wisdom! By following these seven steps, you can start using Amish herbal remedies in a way that fits into your life.

Step 1: Assess Your Personal Health Needs

Before you begin using herbal remedies, it's important to understand your unique health needs. Taking the time to assess your overall well-being will help you choose the right herbs and treatments. This step is about observing, reflecting, and getting to know your body better. Here's how to get started:

1. **Reflect on Your Current Health**

    Begin by asking yourself some simple yet meaningful questions:

- How do I feel most days? Do I have a lot of energy, or do I feel drained?
- Do I struggle with specific issues like stress, poor sleep, or frequent digestive discomfort?
- Are there recurring problems, such as seasonal allergies, headaches, or skin irritations?

Identifying these patterns will give you a clearer idea of what areas to focus on.

2. **Keep a Health Journal**

Write your observations down in a journal. Even a few notes each day can go a long way in spotting trends. For instance:

- Record how you feel in the morning, afternoon, and evening.
- Note how symptoms like fatigue, tension, or bloating appear and when they're most intense.
- Look for triggers. Are you more stressed after a long workday? Does a lack of sleep make you feel worse?

Your journal is a tool to help track ongoing progress and changes.

3. **Identify Short-Term and Long-Term Goals**

Set some health goals for yourself. Divide them into two categories:

- ***Short-term goals:*** These are smaller issues you'd like to tackle sooner, like relieving stress, improving digestion, or sleeping better. Herbs like chamomile or peppermint could help here.
- ***Long-term goals:*** Are there chronic issues you'd like to address, such as improving immunity to reduce colds or managing inflammation? Remedies like echinacea or consistent herbal use may fit into this plan.

This sort of planning will guide your choices as you move forward.

4. **Be Honest About Your Lifestyle**

Consider your daily habits and routines. Things like diet, hydration, stress levels, and sleep all affect your physical and mental health. Ask yourself:

- Am I eating nutritious meals or relying too much on processed foods?
- Do I stay hydrated throughout the day?
- Am I taking time for self-care, or do I feel overwhelmed?

Making even small adjustments in your routine can amplify the effects of herbal remedies, enhancing your results.

5. **Consult a Professional**

   If you're unsure about where to begin, seek advice from a healthcare provider or herbalist. They can:

   - Help you identify health needs you might not have noticed.
   - Ensure herbal remedies won't interfere with medications or existing conditions.
   - Suggest herbs and dosages tailored to your goals.

   For example, if you're trying to improve sleep, they might suggest adding chamomile tea to your nightly routine and explain how much to use.

6. **Start Simple**

   You don't need to address everything all at once. Start with a single issue that feels manageable, like reducing stress or improving digestion. Focus on incorporating one or two herbs at a time so you can easily monitor their effects.

By thoroughly assessing your health, you're setting yourself up for success. This foundation lets you choose the remedies that will work best for your unique needs. Remember, the goal isn't perfection but progress.

Step 2: Selecting Appropriate Herbs

Once you understand your health needs, it's time to choose the herbs that suit your goals. This step is all about finding the right match for your body.

1. **Learn About Commonly Used Herbs**

    Start by exploring herbs that are well-known for addressing specific health concerns. To help narrow your focus, here are some popular choices and their benefits:

    - *Echinacea*: Boosts the immune system, helping to prevent and reduce the severity of colds and infections.
    - *Chamomile*: Known for its calming effects, it's great for reducing stress, improving sleep, and soothing an upset stomach.
    - *Peppermint*: Helps with digestion, relieves headaches, eases muscle pain, and can act as a decongestant.
    - *Lavender*: A versatile herb for relaxation, anxiety relief, and improving sleep quality.
    - *Ginger*: Excellent for nausea, digestive issues, and reducing inflammation.

    This list is just a starting point, so feel free to expand your knowledge and explore other herbs that align with your needs.

2. **Do Your Research**

Take some time to dig deeper into the herbs you're curious about. Look for information on their history, medicinal properties, and traditional uses. Here's how to go about it:

- ***Read books or guides on herbal medicine:*** These often provide detailed descriptions of herbs and their effects.
- ***Join online herbal communities:*** Forums and discussion groups can offer helpful tips and personal experiences.
- ***Visit trusted websites:*** Focus on platforms that are backed by herbalists or health professionals.

Tip: Remember, not all sources are reliable. Cross-check information to ensure accuracy.

3. **Match Herbs to Your Needs**

Once you've learned more about herbs, align them with your health goals. For example:

- If you want better immunity, consider echinacea or elderberry.
- For better sleep and relaxation, chamomile and lavender are excellent choices.
- If digestion is an issue, peppermint or ginger can be very helpful.

You may find that multiple herbs could meet your needs. That's okay! Start simple, and pick one or two to try first.

4. **Experiment Gradually**

   When using herbs for the first time, approach it like an experiment:

   - Begin with small amounts. For example, drink one cup of herbal tea or use one drop of tincture to see how your body responds.
   - Monitor the effects. Does the herb make you feel better? Do you notice any side effects?

   This trial-and-error approach helps you learn what works for your unique body.

5. **Understand Potential Interactions**

   Herbs are natural, but they're still powerful. It's important to know how they might interact with medications or preexisting health conditions. For example:

   - Echinacea might not be suitable for people with autoimmune disorders.
   - Chamomile, while gentle, may cause allergic reactions in those sensitive to ragweed.

- St. John's Wort, a common herb for mood enhancement, can interfere with birth control pills and other medications.

If you're unsure about an herb's suitability, consult a healthcare provider or herbalist.

6. **Think About Forms of Herbs**

   Herbs can be used in different ways depending on your preference and lifestyle. Understanding these forms can make it easier to choose one that fits:

   Teas: Easy to prepare and enjoy daily. Great for calming herbs like chamomile or peppermint.

   Tinctures: Concentrated liquid extracts that are fast-acting and long-lasting.

   Capsules: Convenient for those who don't like the flavor of certain herbs.

   Essential oils: Best for topical use or aromatherapy to enhance relaxation.

   Pick a form that works best for your routine and needs.

7. **Consult Herbal Experts**

   If you're feeling unsure or overwhelmed, don't hesitate to ask for help. Herbalists are trained to guide you in selecting the right remedies. They can provide insights into herbal combinations, dosing, and usage specific to your health concerns.

Selecting the right herbs is an empowering part of your natural health journey. By taking your time to research, experimenting with small amounts, and understanding interactions, you can confidently introduce herbs into your life.

Step 3: Sourcing Quality Ingredients

When it comes to herbal remedies, the quality of your ingredients can make all the difference. High-quality herbs ensure that you get the maximum health benefits and avoid potential contaminants. Here's how you can source the best herbs for your needs, whether you grow them yourself or purchase them from trusted suppliers.

1. **Grow Your Own Herbs**

    One of the best ways to ensure quality is to grow herbs yourself. It's more affordable in the long run, and you'll have full control over how they're cultivated. Here's how to get started:

    - *Choose beginner-friendly herbs*: If you're new to gardening, start with easy-to-grow plants like peppermint, chamomile, or basil.
    - *Use organic soil*: Healthy soil provides the foundation for strong, nutrient-rich herbs. Opt

for organic potting mix and avoid synthetic pesticides or fertilizers.
- **Pick the right spot**: Most herbs thrive in sunny locations with well-draining soil. Make sure your garden or pots receive 6–8 hours of sunlight daily.
- **Harvest at the right time**: For optimal potency, harvest herbs when they're mature but before they start flowering (with some exceptions like chamomile). Early morning is often the best time to do this, as the essential oils are most concentrated.

Growing your own herbs is not only rewarding but also guarantees freshness and purity.

2. **Buy Locally**

Supporting local farmers is another excellent way to source fresh, high-quality herbs. Here's what to keep in mind:

- **Visit farmers' markets**: Local vendors often sell fresh, organic herbs that are recently harvested. Chat with them about their growing practices to ensure no harmful chemicals are used.
- **Check for freshness**: Look for vibrant, brightly colored leaves with a strong, fresh aroma.

Avoid anything that looks wilted, yellowed, or dried out.

- *Ask about the source*: Many farmers are happy to share how they grow and harvest their plants. Don't hesitate to ask about their methods to ensure transparency.

Buying herbs locally not only supports small businesses but also shortens the time between harvest and use, ensuring peak freshness.

3. **Shop From Reputable Suppliers**

If growing your own or buying locally isn't an option, you can still find high-quality herbs online or in specialty stores. Here's how to make sure you get the best:

- *Look for organic certification*: Opt for suppliers that sell USDA-certified organic herbs, as these are grown without harmful pesticides or synthetic fertilizers.
- *Choose transparent brands*: Reputable suppliers provide detailed information about the sourcing of their products. Look for companies that list the country of origin and their testing process for purity.

- ***Read reviews***: Customer feedback can give you valuable insight into a supplier's quality and reliability.
- ***Prioritize freshness***: Check the packaging date. Dried herbs should be vibrant in color and aromatic, even if stored in sealed bags or jars. Avoid anything that looks dull, faded, or dusty.

Some specialized herbal shops also sell tinctures, essential oils, and capsules, which are convenient if you're looking for ready-to-use forms of herbs.

4. **Avoid Harmful Chemicals**

Whether you're growing, buying locally, or sourcing online, it's crucial to avoid herbs grown with harmful chemicals. Non-organic herbs can be exposed to pesticides or contaminants that may reduce their efficacy or even pose health risks.

- ***For home gardeners:*** Stick to natural pest control methods like neem oil, companion planting, or diatomaceous earth.
- ***For buyers:*** Avoid herbs that have a strong chemical smell or unnaturally shiny leaves, as these could indicate the use of chemical treatments.

5. **Store Herbs Properly**

   Once you've sourced high-quality herbs, proper storage will keep them fresh and potent for longer.

   - *For fresh herbs:* Store them in the refrigerator with the stems placed in a glass of water and loosely covered with a plastic bag.
   - *For dried herbs:* Keep them in airtight containers away from light, heat, and moisture to preserve their potency.
   - *For bulk herbs:* Monitor them regularly to ensure they aren't exposed to humidity, pests, or mold growth.

Sourcing high-quality herbs is a critical step in creating effective and safe remedies. Whether you grow them yourself, buy locally, or order from trusted suppliers, focus on freshness, organic practices, and transparency. With a little effort, you'll have top-notch ingredients that offer maximum healing potential.

Step 4: Preparing Remedies

Once you've sourced high-quality herbs, the next step is to turn them into remedies tailored to your needs. While the methods for creating herbal teas, tinctures, salves, and infusions were covered earlier, this step focuses on the environment and mindset needed to make the process smooth, satisfying, and effective.

1. **Why Preparation Matters**

   The way you prepare your remedies plays a big role in their effectiveness. Properly prepared remedies ensure that the herbs maintain their potency and deliver the benefits you're seeking. It's not just about "getting it done" but doing it with care and intention. Taking the time to create an organized and clean setup not only adds to the remedies' quality but also makes the experience more enjoyable and rewarding.

2. **Organize Your Workspace**

   Having a dedicated and well-organized space for preparing your herbal remedies can make the process easier and more efficient. Here are some tips to get started:

   - *Choose a Clean Surface*: Use a clean, flat surface in a quiet corner of your kitchen or workspace. Ideally, this should be away from distractions and clutter.
   - *Gather Your Tools*: Keep items like jars, straining equipment, measuring spoons, and utensils within easy reach. Store them in a designated drawer or container so you're not hunting for tools when you start.
   - *Create Labels in Advance*: Write out the herb names, dates, and storage instructions beforehand to keep everything organized.

Having pre-made labels saves time and helps avoid confusion.
- *Use a Tray or Basket for Supplies*: Group your herbs and tools in baskets or trays so they're easy to transport and keep together.

3. **Ensure Cleanliness**

Cleanliness is crucial when working with herbal remedies to avoid contamination and preserve the herbs' healing properties. Here's how to maintain a clean and safe workspace:

- *Wash Your Hands*: Always wash your hands thoroughly before handling herbs or tools.
- *Sterilize Containers*: Boil glass jars, bottles, and utensils to sterilize them before use. This step keeps bacteria, mold, or other impurities from spoiling your remedies.
- *Avoid Cross-Contamination*: Assign specific tools like cutting boards or spoons for herbal use only, especially if preparing multiple remedies.
- *Wipe Surfaces*: Regularly clean and sanitize your workspace before and after making remedies.

4. **Create a Preparation Routine**

Having a routine makes preparing remedies feel less overwhelming, especially when you're just starting out.

Establishing consistent steps can also help you stay organized and enjoy the process.

- ***Dedicate Time Each Week***: Set aside an hour or two each week to prepare your remedies. Treat it as self-care time where you can slow down and focus on your health.
- ***Start Small***: Don't feel pressured to make multiple remedies at once. Begin with one or two that address your priorities, and expand gradually as you gain confidence.
- ***Keep Notes***: Record the herbs you use, the methods you try, and how each remedy turns out. This "herbal journal" will help you refine your techniques over time.
- ***Store Strategically***: Once your remedies are ready, store them in clearly labeled containers and keep them in designated spots (e.g., tinctures in a cabinet, teas in airtight tins). This reduces chaos in your storage area and keeps your remedies fresh.

5. **Bring Intention to the Process**

Preparing remedies can become a mindful and almost meditative practice. Approach each step with care and appreciation for the natural ingredients you're working with. Light a candle, play calming music, or simply enjoy the quiet moment. This mindful approach not only enhances the experience but deepens your connection with the remedies you're creating.

Good preparation goes beyond following recipes; it's about creating a system that works for you while ensuring the potency, hygiene, and organization of your remedies. When your workspace is set up and your routine is established, the process becomes a relaxing ritual rather than a chore.

Step 5: Integrating Remedies into Daily Routines

Now that you've prepared your remedies, it's time to make them a natural part of your day. Incorporating herbal remedies into your daily routine can feel seamless and enjoyable with a few mindful strategies. The key is to pair your remedies with activities you're already doing and to build habits gradually so they stick.

1. **Start Small and Simple**

    Building new habits takes time, so don't feel pressured to overhaul your entire day all at once. Begin with one or two remedies that address your most immediate health goals and integrate them into your current routines. For example:

- *Mornings*: Start your day with an energizing cup of herbal tea, such as nettle or peppermint, to wake up your body naturally.
- *Evenings*: Add a few drops of a calming tincture like valerian root into your bedtime ritual to promote restful sleep.

By starting small, you'll have a higher chance of sticking with your new habits and feeling the benefits over time.

2. **Pair Remedies with Existing Routines**

One of the easiest ways to remember to use your remedies is to connect them with things you already do every day. This simple "habit stacking" approach ensures that taking your remedies doesn't feel like an extra task. Here are some ideas:

- *With Meals*: Take herbal tinctures that support digestion (such as ginger or fennel) before or after eating.
- *After a Shower*: Use soothing herbal salves, like calendula or lavender, after your shower to lock in moisture and care for your skin.
- *At Your Desk*: Keep small jars of herbal tea blends within arm's reach at work so you can brew a cup during breaks to stay hydrated and focused.

When remedies are part of something familiar, they'll feel like a natural extension of your day.

3. **Create Rituals Around Your Remedies**

   Herbal remedies often work best when they're approached with intention and mindfulness. By turning their use into a mini ritual, you'll be more likely to enjoy the process and stick with it. For instance:

   - *Herbal Tea Time*: Dedicate 10–15 minutes to savoring your tea instead of rushing through it. Pair this time with quietly reading, journaling, or reflecting on your day.
   - *Tincture Rituals*: Set a specific time of the day to take your tinctures consistently. Place the tincture bottle near your coffee maker, toothbrush, or other visual cue to remind you.
   - *Nighttime Comfort*: Use salves or balms as part of a calming nighttime routine. Massage them into your skin while taking deep breaths to unwind before bed.

   Rituals help elevate the practice from a simple task to a meaningful moment of self-care.

4. **Use Visual Reminders**

   When starting a new habit, visual cues work wonders in keeping you on track. Strategically place your remedies in spots where you'll see them throughout the day:

- **On the Kitchen Counter**: Keep your teas, tinctures, or infused oils neatly displayed where you prepare meals so you won't forget.
- **By Your Bedside**: Store any nighttime remedies, like a relaxing lavender spray or sleep tincture, next to your alarm clock or lamp.
- **On Your Work Desk**: Place a small dish with your salves or creams on your desk so you can apply them during a break.

Seeing your remedies often creates gentle reminders to use them.

5. Build a Consistent Schedule

Consistency is key for herbal remedies to be effective. Consider creating a schedule that works with your lifestyle. For example:

- **Morning Routine**: Start your day with an herbal tea or infusion to boost your energy and support overall wellness.
- **Afternoon Pick-Me-Up**: Use a mentally refreshing remedy like a rosemary salve or a few drops of lemon balm tincture mid-day to stay alert.

- ***Evening Wind-Down***: Incorporate remedies that promote relaxation during your evening routine, such as a chamomile-infused tea or warm bath with herbal oils.

When you anchor your remedies to specific times, they become as automatic as brushing your teeth.

6. **Track Your Progress**

    If you're trying out multiple remedies, it's helpful to track what works for you. Use a health journal to note:

    - Which remedies you used.
    - The times or situations you used them.
    - How they made you feel.

    Over time, this record will help you refine your routine and understand which remedies best meet your needs.

7. **Include the Family**

    If you live with others, get them involved in your herbal routine. Herbal remedies like teas and salves often benefit the whole household. Make it social by sharing a calming tea before bed or giving each other small salve massages to relieve tension after a long day.

Integrating herbal remedies into your daily life doesn't have to feel like a chore. By starting small, pairing remedies with existing habits, and creating meaningful rituals, you'll find that they enhance not just your health, but your overall sense of well-being. Think of this step as an opportunity to intentionally slow down and care for yourself in small but powerful ways.

Step 6: Monitoring and Documenting Effects

Once you've integrated herbal remedies into your routine, the next vital step is to monitor their effects and track your progress. This ensures you're using the remedies effectively and allows you to make adjustments as needed. Since herbal remedies often work gradually, documenting your experience can help you identify patterns, celebrate improvements, and fine-tune your regimen.

1. **The Importance of Monitoring**

    Herbal remedies often take time to show noticeable changes. Unlike instant fixes, their benefits build up over consistent use. Monitoring helps you recognize the subtle shifts in your health that might otherwise go unnoticed. Are you sleeping better? Do you feel calmer or more energized? These small victories can validate your efforts and keep you motivated.

    Additionally, paying attention to how your body responds can help you detect any negative reactions or identify remedies that may not suit you. This awareness is key to ensuring the safe and effective use of herbs.

2. Keeping a Health Journal

A health journal is a simple yet powerful way to document your experience with herbal remedies. It doesn't have to be fancy; a notebook, an app, or even a spreadsheet can do the trick. Here's what to include:

- ***The Remedies You're Using***: Write down the name, type (tea, tincture, etc.), and dosage of each remedy.
- ***When and How You Take Them***: Note the time of day and whether you take the remedy with food, on an empty stomach, or as part of a specific routine.
- ***Your Symptoms or Concerns***: Record the health issue you're addressing, such as stress, poor sleep, or digestion troubles.
- ***Daily Observations***: Jot down any changes you notice, even if they seem minor. Improvements or new symptoms might take a few days to become apparent.

For example, "Started taking valerian tincture for sleep on Monday night. Slept deeper and woke up feeling rested." Over time, these notes will reveal patterns and insights.

3. **Noting Changes in Symptoms**

   When documenting effects, it's important to pay attention to both physical and emotional changes. Herbs often affect the whole body, so even if your primary concern improves, you may notice benefits in other areas too. Here's what to evaluate:

   - *Energy Levels*: Are you feeling more alert or fatigued?
   - *Mood Shifts*: Do you feel calmer, more focused, or less irritable?
   - *Symptom Relief*: Has your digestion improved? Are headaches or joint pain less frequent?
   - *Sleep Patterns*: Are you falling asleep faster and staying asleep longer?

   To make tracking easier, you might use a simple rating system, like a 1–10 scale, to rate how you're feeling before and after taking remedies. For example, rate your stress levels in the evening before taking a tincture and again the next morning.

4. **Identifying Patterns Over Time**

   While some herbal remedies deliver quick results, others require consistency to show their full effects. That's why it's helpful to review your journal every couple of weeks or at the end of each month. Look for trends such as:

- Gradual improvement in symptoms.
- Specific remedies that seem especially effective.
- Remedies that don't appear to make a noticeable difference.

For instance, if you notice that your energy consistently dips in the afternoon, you may consider adding a mid-day infusion of energizing herbs like ginseng or nettle. Conversely, if a remedy isn't working after a fair trial period, it might be time to adjust the dosage or explore alternatives.

5. **Be Patient and Consistent**

It's important to approach the process with patience. Herbal remedies are not quick fixes but rather tools to support long-term health. Stick with your regimen for 4–6 weeks before making major changes unless you experience adverse effects. Use this time to allow the herbs to interact naturally with your body.

If you're feeling stuck or unsure, revisit your goals. What were you hoping to achieve when you started using these remedies? Reflecting on your "why" can provide reassurance and help you stay consistent.

6. **When to Seek Professional Advice**

   While many herbs are safe for self-guided use, consulting with a healthcare professional can provide valuable insights. If you're not seeing desired results, consider speaking with an herbalist, naturopath, or other qualified professional. Bring your health journal to the appointment so they can better understand your experiences and recommend adjustments.

   Additionally, if you experience unexpected side effects, stop using the remedy immediately and seek guidance. Some reactions may be due to improper dosage, herb-drug interactions, or individual sensitivities.

7. **Staying Engaged in the Process**

   Tracking your progress doesn't have to feel like work. Here are some tips to make it more enjoyable:

   - ***Celebrate Small Wins***: Acknowledge any progress you make, even if it feels minor. Healing is a journey, and every step counts.
   - ***Make Journaling a Ritual***: Pair it with a relaxing activity like sipping tea or listening to music at the end of the day.
   - ***Get Creative***: Use drawings, stickers, or color coding in your journal to make it visually appealing.

Monitoring and documenting the effects of herbal remedies allows you to take an active role in your health. By carefully tracking your experiences, you'll not only gain a deeper understanding of your body but also build confidence in using herbs effectively.

Step 7: Adjusting and Customizing Your Approach

The final step in incorporating Amish herbal remedies into your life is all about personalization. Once you've spent time monitoring how your body responds to different remedies, it's time to refine your approach.

Everyone is unique, and your herbal routine should reflect your individual needs, preferences, lifestyle, and even the changing seasons. This is where herbalism becomes as much an art as it is a science, and the process is both empowering and rewarding.

1. **The Power of Flexibility**

   Herbal remedies aren't a one-size-fits-all solution, and that's part of their beauty. What works perfectly for one person may need tweaking for another. By staying open to change and actively listening to your body, you can fine-tune your remedies to work best for you.

   For example, you might find that a lower dose of a calming tincture works better for you than the suggested amount, or that switching herbs seasonally boosts their effectiveness. Flexibility ensures your herbal practice evolves as your needs do.

2. Experimenting with Dosages

One of the easiest ways to customize your remedies is through adjusting dosages. Start low and go slow. Many herbal remedies are just as effective in smaller amounts, so you may not need the "standard" quantity listed on your tincture bottle. Pay attention to how your body feels, and tweak the amount to suit your personal tolerance and needs.

For example:

- If an energizing herbal tea feels too stimulating, reduce the amount of herbs used per cup or steep it for a shorter time.
- If a remedy feels only partially effective, consider increasing the dosage slightly while ensuring you stay within safe limits.

Keep notes in your health journal as you experiment, so you can track which adjustments work best.

3. Combining Remedies for Better Results

Sometimes, a combination of herbs can amplify the benefits you're seeking. This approach is called creating a synergistic blend, where multiple herbs work together to achieve a holistic effect.

For instance:

- If you're addressing stress and poor sleep, you might pair a calming tea like chamomile with a valerian tincture for a more comprehensive approach.
- For immune support during colder months, combine herbs like elderberry, echinacea, and ginger into one remedy.

Experiment with different combinations, but take care to research any potential interactions between herbs or consult with a professional before mixing.

4. **Adapting to Seasonal Needs**

Your body's needs can change with the seasons, and your herbal remedies should adapt accordingly. Herbs that support you in the heat of summer might not address the challenges of cold winter months, and vice versa.

Here are some seasonal examples to consider:

Spring: Focus on detoxifying and energizing herbs like dandelion root or nettle to support your body's natural renewal process.

Summer: Hydrating herbs like hibiscus or peppermint can help you stay cool and refreshed.

Fall: Support your immune system with herbs such as elderberry or astragalus as the weather changes.

Winter: Turn to warming, circulation-boosting herbs like cinnamon, ginger, or turmeric to combat the chill and improve digestion.

Seasonal adjustments can renew your routine and keep your remedies aligned with what your body needs at any given time.

5. **Lifestyle Adjustments and Customization**

   Major life changes, such as starting a new job, becoming a parent, or dealing with increased physical activity, can impact your health. Your herbal remedies should adapt to fit these changes.

   <u>For example:</u>

   - If you've started a demanding job, you might add adaptogenic herbs like ashwagandha for stress support.
   - If you've taken up rigorous exercise, consider anti-inflammatory remedies like turmeric or arnica to aid muscle recovery.
   - If you're traveling often, immune-boosting remedies like echinacea or elderberry can help

fend off common colds from long flights or new environments.

Additionally, consider how your preferences play a role in customization. If you dislike the taste of a particular herb, explore other forms like capsules or infused oils. There's no wrong way to use herbs as long as they're effective and enjoyable for you.

6. Learning to Listen to Your Body

The most important step in customizing your herbal approach is tuning in to what your body is telling you. Think of your body as a partner in this process. If a remedy doesn't seem to work or starts feeling ineffective over time, don't be afraid to take a break, try a new herb, or re-evaluate your goals. Remember, your needs will likely shift as you grow and change.

7. Knowing When to Adjust or Stop

Sometimes, your herbal regimen might need a major adjustment or even to be paused. Be mindful of these signs:

- The remedy feels too strong or causes discomfort.
- You've reached your desired health outcome and no longer need the remedy as frequently.

- A remedy loses effectiveness after long-term use (this can happen with certain herbs).
- Honoring these cues ensures you're using herbs in a balanced and sustainable way.

Step 7 is all about taking ownership of your herbal practice and making it uniquely yours. By adjusting dosages, experimenting with blends, and adapting to life's changes, you're creating a health routine that's as flexible and dynamic as you are. Trust your instincts, stay curious, and enjoy the process of evolving your practice.

Sample Recipes for Common Ailments

Below are some sample recipes to get you started on your herbal journey. These are just a taste of the many possibilities and combinations that exist within herbalism. Feel free to adjust ingredients and dosages as needed for your individual needs.

Herbal Tea Blends for Colds and Flu

Elderberry Immune Boost Tea

Ingredients:

- 1 tbsp dried elderberries
- 1 tsp echinacea leaves
- 1 tsp dried ginger root
- 1 tsp honey (optional)
- 2 cups water

Instructions:

1. Boil water in a small pot.
2. Add elderberries, echinacea, and ginger. Simmer for 10 minutes.
3. Strain into a mug and sweeten with honey if desired.

Benefits: Elderberries boost immunity, echinacea reduces cold symptoms, and ginger fights inflammation while soothing sore throats.

Peppermint Eucalyptus Breath Easy Tea

Ingredients:

- 1 tsp dried peppermint leaves
- 1 tsp dried eucalyptus leaves
- Juice of ½ lemon
- 1 tsp honey
- 1 cup boiling water

Instructions:

1. Place peppermint and eucalyptus leaves in a mug.
2. Add boiling water and steep for 5-7 minutes.
3. Strain, then add lemon juice and honey.

Benefits: This tea clears nasal passages, soothes coughs, and supports respiratory health during colds.

Lemon Ginger Detox Tea

Ingredients:

- 1 tsp dried ginger root
- 1 tsp dried lemon peel
- 1 tsp chamomile flowers
- 1 cup boiling water

Instructions:

1. Steep all ingredients in boiling water for 8-10 minutes.
2. Strain and enjoy warm.

Benefits: Eases congestion, boosts detoxification, and promotes relaxation to aid recovery.

Spiced Immunity Tea

Ingredients:

- 1 tsp turmeric powder
- ½ tsp cinnamon powder
- ½ tsp dried cloves
- 1 tbsp honey
- 1 cup almond or oat milk

Instructions:

1. Heat milk over low heat without boiling.
2. Stir in turmeric, cinnamon, cloves, and honey until combined.
3. Serve warm as a comforting evening drink.

Benefits: Rich in antioxidants, this tea reduces inflammation and strengthens immunity.

Cold Comfort Hibiscus Blend

Ingredients:

- 1 tbsp dried hibiscus flowers
- 1 tsp rosehips
- 1 tsp dried orange peel
- 1 tsp honey
- 1.5 cups water

Instructions:

1. Simmer hibiscus, rosehips, and orange peel in water for 10 minutes.
2. Strain, sweeten with honey, and enjoy.

Benefits: High in vitamin C, this tea soothes sore throats and bolsters immune function.

Soothing Salves for Aches and Pains

Arnica Muscle Relief Salve

Ingredients:

- 1 cup arnica-infused olive oil
- 1 oz beeswax
- Optional: 5 drops peppermint essential oil

Instructions:

1. Melt the beeswax in a double boiler.
2. Stir in the arnica oil and optional essential oil.
3. Pour into tins or jars and cool until solid.

Benefits: Arnica soothes muscle pain, while peppermint provides a cooling effect.

Calendula Healing Balm

Ingredients:

- 1 cup calendula-infused oil
- 1 oz beeswax
- Optional: 5 drops lavender essential oil

Instructions:

1. Combine calendula-infused oil and beeswax in a double boiler until melted.
2. Stir well and pour into containers.
3. Allow to cool and solidify.

Benefits: Calendula reduces inflammation, eases soreness, and promotes skin healing.

St. John's Wort Nerve Pain Balm

Ingredients:

- 1 cup St. John's Wort-infused oil
- 1 oz beeswax
- Optional: 5 drops eucalyptus essential oil

Instructions:

1. Melt beeswax and combine with St. John's Wort oil in a double boiler.
2. Add eucalyptus oil, stir, and pour into jars to cool.

Benefits: This salve is effective for nerve pain and sore or inflamed joints.

Comfrey Joint Salve

Ingredients:

- 1 cup comfrey-infused oil
- 1 oz beeswax
- Optional: 5 drops rosemary essential oil

Instructions:

1. Heat beeswax and comfrey oil in a double boiler until blended.
2. Mix in essential oil (if desired) and pour into containers.

Benefits: Comfrey supports healing of sprains, bruises, and joint pain.

Ginger Warming Salve

Ingredients:

- 1 cup ginger-infused oil
- 1 oz beeswax
- Optional: 5 drops cinnamon essential oil

Instructions:

1. Melt beeswax and mix with ginger oil.
2. Add essential oil if desired, and pour into tins.

Benefits: Great for cold weather, this salve improves circulation and eases tight muscles.

Natural Solutions for Digestive Issues

Peppermint Fennel Digestive Tea

Ingredients:

- 1 tsp dried peppermint leaves
- 1 tsp fennel seeds
- 1 tsp dried chamomile flowers
- 1 cup boiling water

Instructions:

1. Combine all ingredients in a mug and steep for 7-10 minutes.
2. Strain and enjoy after meals.

Benefits: Relieves bloating, gas, and indigestion.

Ginger Turmeric Stomach-Settler Drink

Ingredients:

- 1 tsp grated fresh ginger
- ½ tsp turmeric powder
- Juice of ½ lemon
- 1 cup warm water

Instructions:

1. Mix all ingredients in warm water.
2. Stir and sip slowly.

Benefits: Reduces nausea and soothes stomach discomfort.

Caraway-Coriander Digestive Blend

Ingredients:

1 tsp caraway seeds

1 tsp coriander seeds

1 cup boiling water

Instructions:

1. Lightly crush seeds and steep them in boiling water for 10 minutes.
2. Strain and drink warm.

Benefits: Helps alleviate gas and enhances digestion.

Licorice Root Digestive Calm Tea

Ingredients:

- 1 tsp dried licorice root
- 1 tsp dried peppermint leaves
- 1 cup boiling water

Instructions:

1. Steep licorice root and peppermint in boiling water for 10 minutes.
2. Strain and enjoy warm.

Benefits: Calms an upset stomach and soothes acid reflux.

Apple Cider Vinegar Herbal Tonic

Ingredients:

- 1 tbsp apple cider vinegar
- 1 tsp dried ginger powder
- 1 tsp honey
- 1 cup warm water

Instructions:

1. Combine all ingredients in a cup of warm water.
2. Stir well and sip slowly.

Benefits: Improves digestion by balancing stomach acid and reducing bloating.

These recipes are simple enough for beginners and showcase the beauty of traditional herbal remedies.

Safety Considerations and Best Practices for Using Amish Herbal Remedies

When it comes to herbal remedies, safety should always come first. While natural, plant-based solutions offer numerous benefits, they must be used responsibly to ensure positive outcomes. Below are important considerations and best practices to help you use Amish herbal remedies effectively and safely.

Understanding Potential Side Effects

Even though herbal remedies come from plants, they are not free from the possibility of side effects. People can react differently to the same herb due to their unique biology, sensitivities, and underlying health conditions.

Common Side Effects

- Mild Allergic Reactions: This might include itching, a rash, or respiratory discomfort. Herbs like chamomile

(related to ragweed) and echinacea can occasionally trigger allergies.
- Digestive Upset: Some herbs, like garlic or ginger, may cause stomach discomfort if consumed in large amounts.
- Headaches or Dizziness: Overuse of certain herbs, such as peppermint or ginseng, may lead to mild headaches or feelings of lightheadedness.

Recognizing Serious Reactions

Pay close attention to how your body responds when introducing a new herbal remedy. Signs of a more severe reaction include:

- Intense swelling or difficulty breathing (seek immediate medical attention).
- Severe gastrointestinal distress.
- Persistent symptoms like headaches or skin rashes.

Best Practices for Avoiding Side Effects

- *Start Small:* Use small doses, such as half a cup of tea or a single drop of tincture, when trying a new herb. Increase dosage gradually while monitoring your body's reaction.
- *Test One Herb at a Time:* If you're trying herbal blends, especially homemade ones, start by testing the individual herbs first. This helps you identify which herb may cause a reaction if discomfort arises.

- *Avoid Long-Term Overuse:* Some herbs, like valerian, should not be used continuously for extended periods. Take breaks to avoid building tolerance or experiencing adverse effects.

If you do experience side effects, stop using the herb immediately and consult a healthcare professional if symptoms persist.

Consulting with Healthcare Professionals

While herbal remedies are natural, they can still interact with medications or exacerbate certain medical conditions. Consulting a doctor ensures you're making safe and informed choices.

When It's Essential to Seek Medical Advice

- *Pre-Existing Conditions:* If you have chronic conditions such as diabetes, high blood pressure, or kidney disease, some herbs may interfere with your health or medications. For example, licorice root may raise blood pressure.
- *Pregnancy and Breastfeeding:* Herbs like nettle or raspberry leaf can be beneficial during pregnancy in moderation, but others like pennyroyal may be harmful. Always check with your doctor before using herbal remedies during these stages.
- *Medications:* Some herbs can amplify or counteract the effects of medications. For instance, St. John's

Wort may weaken the effectiveness of birth control pills or antidepressants.
- *Children and the Elderly:* These groups often have more sensitive systems and may require adjusted doses or avoidance of certain strong herbs, such as ginseng.

How to Approach the Conversation
- *Be Honest:* Share details of the herbal remedies you plan to use, including the specific herbs, quantities, and preparation methods.
- *Bring References:* If you're following a particular recipe or guide, bring it with you to show the healthcare provider exactly what you intend to use.
- *Ask Direct Questions:* For example, ask if a specific herb might interact with your current medication or if it's appropriate for your condition.
- *Respect Their Expertise:* Even if you are passionate about herbal remedies, remember that a doctor's insight is invaluable when it comes to safety and avoiding harm.

Remember, consulting a professional doesn't diminish the value of traditional remedies—in fact, it enhances their effectiveness by ensuring they're used in a medically sound way.

Responsible Use of Herbal Remedies

Responsible use ensures that your remedies are as safe and effective as possible. Whether you're new to herbal medicine or experienced in Amish remedies, following these tips can help you practice with care.

Proper Dosages

- *Follow Guidelines:* Many herbs have specific dosing recommendations. For instance, peppermint tea is often safe at 1–2 cups per day, but drinking excessive amounts can lead to nausea.
- *Listen to Your Body:* If you notice subtle discomfort, such as bloating or headaches, reduce the dosage or stop use altogether.
- *Avoid Overuse:* Herbs are not a "more is better" solution. Using large amounts may overwhelm your body or cause unnecessary strain. Stick to moderate doses.

Understanding Interactions

- *Check for Conflicts:* Research or ask a professional whether an herb could interact with medications, supplements, or other herbs you're currently using. For instance, blood-thinning herbs like ginkgo biloba may interact with prescribed blood thinners.
- *Space Out Usage:* If using both herbs and pharmaceuticals, give your body time to process each.

For example, drink herbal tea a few hours before or after taking medications.

Sourcing High-Quality Herbs

The quality of the herbs you use directly affects the safety and efficacy of your remedies.

- *Buy Organic*: Choose herbs labeled as organic and pesticide-free to avoid contaminants.
- *Avoid Unknown Sources*: Ingredients from unverified sellers may contain impurities or lack potency.
- *Grow Your Own*: Cultivating herbs yourself ensures purity and allows you to keep a close eye on the growing process.

Following Preparation Guidelines

- *Label Remedies Clearly*: Include preparation dates and expiry dates on tinctures, oils, and teas to avoid using expired products.
- *Store Properly*: Keep remedies in airtight containers, away from sunlight and moisture, to maintain their potency.
- *Keeping Records*: Maintain a journal of the herbs you use, the dosage, and any effects you notice. This is not only helpful for monitoring your progress but also valuable if you need to discuss your herbal regimen with a doctor.

Amish herbal remedies are a time-honored way to support your health, but they require mindfulness and respect. By understanding potential side effects, consulting with professionals, and using herbs responsibly, you can enjoy the full benefits of this natural approach to wellness. Taking the time to educate yourself and implement these practices allows you to connect with herbal traditions safely and confidently.

Integrating Amish Remedies with Modern Wellness

Bringing together the time-tested wisdom of Amish herbal remedies and contemporary wellness practices is a powerful way to create a balanced and holistic approach to health. While traditional remedies honor natural healing and simplicity, modern health trends focus on advancing mindfulness, physical fitness, and personalized nutrition.

These two approaches complement each other beautifully, offering you a well-rounded path to living a healthier and more intentional life.

Combining Traditional Wisdom with Modern Practices

The essence of Amish herbal remedies is deeply rooted in nature, simplicity, and self-sufficiency. These time-tested remedies, passed down through generations, offer a natural and effective foundation for supporting health and well-being.

By integrating these traditional practices with modern techniques like yoga, meditation, and personalized diet plans, you can create a balanced approach to wellness that fits seamlessly into your everyday life.

For example:

- Start your day with an energizing herbal tea like nettle or dandelion to gently detoxify your body and boost your energy levels. Pair it with a mid-morning yoga session to feel refreshed, grounded, and ready to take on the day with clarity and focus.
- For relaxation and stress relief, combine calming chamomile tea or a valerian tincture with a mindfulness meditation session. These gentle herbs can help calm your nervous system, making it easier to center your thoughts and manage daily stressors.
- After a long workout or a physically demanding day, soothe sore muscles with herbal salves like calendula or arnica. These natural remedies help reduce inflammation and promote faster recovery, allowing you to stay active and pain-free.

By blending the timeless wisdom of herbal remedies with the innovation of modern wellness practices, you create a synergy that amplifies the benefits of both approaches. This holistic combination not only supports your physical health but also nurtures your mental and emotional well-being, helping you build a lifestyle that is sustainable, balanced, and empowering.

Creating a Balanced and Holistic Lifestyle

Blending herbal remedies with modern wellness practices gives you more than just a set of tools for better health. It invites you to adopt a lifestyle that prioritizes harmony, balance, and meaningful intention in every aspect of your day.

By weaving thoughtful practices into your routine, you can transform the way you care for yourself, making wellness a natural and uplifting part of your life. Here's how you can cultivate this holistic approach:

1. **Intentional Living**

   Living intentionally means being mindful about your choices and actions. Instead of rushing through tasks, pause to focus on their deeper purpose and how they contribute to your overall well-being. Herbal remedies are perfect companions for this mindset.

   <u>For example:</u>

   - When preparing herbal tea, take a moment to appreciate the aroma, color, and warmth it brings. Reflect on the nurturing qualities of the herbs and how they support your body.
   - During your morning routine, include moments of gratitude—for the nourishing food you eat, the remedies you take, or simply the breath of a new day.

Intentional living doesn't require drastic changes. Simple shifts, like preparing meals consciously or journaling your thoughts, can ground you in the moment and bring greater meaning to your routines.

2. **Self-Care as a Ritual**

Transform your daily wellness habits into cherished rituals. Self-care isn't selfish; it's an act of love toward yourself. When you approach these moments with reverence and care, even everyday tasks can feel restorative.

Here are some ways to turn self-care into a ritual:

- *Making Herbal Remedies*: Treat the process of preparing a salve, tincture, or tea as a moment of mindfulness. Play calming music, light a candle, and enjoy the creative act of healing.
- *Evening Wind-Down*: End your day with a calming ritual like sipping chamomile tea with a journal or enjoying an herbal bath with soothing lavender and rose petals.
- *Morning Grounding Practices*: Combine a short meditation with a stimulating herbal infusion to energize your day.

The key is to find joy and comfort in these activities. Over time, they'll not only nurture your well-being but also become a soothing respite from daily demands.

3. **Continuous Learning**

    The world of herbal remedies and wellness trends is an exciting space filled with opportunities to grow and adapt. By staying curious and open to new information, you can make better decisions about what works for you and your lifestyle.

    <u>**Here's how to keep learning:**</u>

    - *Explore New Herbs*: Introduce yourself to a single new herb each month. For example, if you've never used ashwagandha or astragalus, try incorporating them into teas or smoothies and learn about their benefits.
    - *Read and Connect*: Seek out books, blogs, videos, or community classes related to herbalism and overall wellness. Engage in conversations with others who share similar interests to expand your knowledge.
    - *Experiment with Trends*: While sticking to what works is important, don't shy away from exploring modern wellness techniques like guided breathwork, sound healing, or nutrient pairing alongside your trusted remedies.

Continuous learning isn't just about adding knowledge; it's about deepening your relationship with your health. Each discovery reinforces the empowering act of taking care of your mind, body, and spirit.

4. Personalization

One size does not fit all, and your wellness routine should reflect your individuality. What makes you feel vibrant, calm, or focused won't necessarily work for someone else, and that's okay. Creating a personalized approach ensures you have something tailored just for you.

Here are some ways to personalize your lifestyle:

- *Tailoring Dosages*: You may find that a smaller dose of a herbal tincture suits you better than the standard recommendation, or that a heavier brew is what your body craves. Learn to fine-tune these remedies based on your needs.
- *Adapting to Preferences*: If you dislike the bitter taste of an herbal tea, try it in capsule form. Prefer cold drinks? Prepare iced infusions in the warmer months instead of hot brews.
- *Reflect Your Goals*: Align your remedies and wellness practices with your current priorities. For instance, if stress reduction is a focus, double down on calming teas, yoga, and quiet

time. If you're working on fitness, focus on remedies that aid recovery and energy, like turmeric or ginseng.

Keep in mind that your needs will shift over time due to seasons, life changes, or simply how your body evolves. Being adaptable and confident in customizing your approach will help your wellness routine grow with you.

Creating a balanced and holistic lifestyle doesn't happen all at once. It blossoms through small, intentional steps that build upon one another. By practicing intentional living, elevating self-care into rituals, committing to lifelong learning, and tailoring your wellness practices to fit you, you create a framework for not just better health, but a more joyful and fulfilling life.

Resources and Further Reading

Exploring Amish herbal remedies offers a doorway into a rich tradition of natural healing. To help you deepen your understanding and expand your practice, here's a curated list of resources, including books, online communities, and opportunities to connect with practitioners. These tools serve as pathways to advance your knowledge and strengthen your herbal wellness routines.

Recommended Books and Publications

Begin your learning with these insightful books that blend traditional Amish wisdom with practical health guidance:

1. ***Amish Herbal and Natural Remedies (Hardcover):*** This book offers a collection of herbal remedies focused on simplicity and natural solutions. From soothing teas to healing salves, it guides you through effective treatments inspired by Amish traditions.

    Here's a link to the book: https://tinyurl.com/4f27aswt.

2. ***Amish Folk Medicine:*** Explore simple home remedies made from everyday ingredients like herbs, foods, and

vitamins. This book is organized by health issue, offering practical tips for common concerns.

Here's a link to the book: https://tinyurl.com/2f37b5e9.

3. ***The Amish Remedies Collection:*** With over 1,300 natural recipes, this guide offers comprehensive insights into family wellness. It includes step-by-step instructions for tinctures, salves, syrups, and teas, making it ideal for beginners and experienced herbalists alike.

   Here's a link to the book: https://tinyurl.com/yxyvcur7.

Online Communities and Workshops

Connecting with like-minded individuals is an excellent way to expand your knowledge and garner support for your herbal practices. Here are some trusted platforms:

1. **American Herbalists Guild (AHG)**

   AHG is a prominent association offering a directory of qualified clinical herbalists, herbalism courses, educational events, and resources to further your learning. Joining their network empowers you with access to a wealth of knowledge.

   Here's a link to the website: https://americanherbalistsguild.com/.

2. **Herbalists Without Borders (HWB)**

   HWB promotes grassroots initiatives like community-supported herbalism, offering free clinics, herbal care kits, and plant-based education. Explore their community projects to connect with others passionate about accessible, natural healthcare.

   Here's a link to the website: https://hwbglobal.org/our-work/community-supported-herbalism/.

Connecting with Practitioners

Engaging with experienced practitioners can be one of the most enriching parts of your herbal wellness journey. These connections provide unique insights and valuable wisdom about traditional remedies that can't always be found in books or online. Here's how to immerse yourself in this community and learn directly from experts:

Seek Out Herbal Workshops and Health Fairs

Workshops and health fairs are fantastic opportunities to meet practitioners and gain hands-on experience with Amish herbal remedies and traditional herbalism.

- *Explore Local Events*: Look for events hosted near Amish communities or in regions that celebrate holistic health. These fairs often feature

demonstrations like brewing herbal teas, crafting salves, or identifying medicinal plants.
- **Sign Up for Specialty Classes**: Many herbalists offer workshops focused on specific remedies or herbs. These are great for gaining in-depth knowledge, particularly if you're interested in learning how to make tinctures, poultices, or herbal tonics from scratch.
- **Attend Seasonal Herb Walks**: Some communities host guided plant identification walks, which are an interactive way to learn about local flora and their medicinal uses.

Participate in Regional Gatherings

Larger gatherings and conferences bring together herbalists from various traditions, including those inspired by Amish practices.

- **Herbal Conferences**: Events like herbal symposiums or wellness expos are excellent places to hear lectures from experienced practitioners. Topics typically range from growing herbs to incorporating remedies into modern healthcare practices.
- **Cultural Festivals**: Amish-focused or rural cultural festivals often feature booths and presentations about traditional health practices, offering a chance to explore remedies specific to their heritage.

- *Networking Opportunities*: These gatherings are not just educational but also social. Strike up conversations with speakers and vendors, ask questions, and exchange contact details to extend your herbalist network.

Build Relationships with AHG and HWB Members

Joining established organizations like the American Herbalists Guild (AHG) and Herbalists Without Borders (HWB) can open doors to a wealth of resources and mentorship opportunities.

- *American Herbalists Guild*: AHG members often include clinical herbalists with years of experience. Visit their directory to find a practitioner near you, and don't hesitate to reach out to them for consultations or advice. AHG also offers webinars, classes, and a robust mentorship program to deepen your skills.
- *Herbalists Without Borders*: HWB focuses on mutual aid and community outreach, making their initiatives accessible to herbal enthusiasts of all levels. Get involved in their community-supported projects, such as creating care packages or working with apothecaries, to learn from practitioners while making a difference.

Additional Tips for Connecting

- *Volunteer or Intern*: Many experienced herbalists or small-scale herbal operations welcome help. Volunteering your time not only provides a deeper understanding but also builds lasting mentorships.
- *Ask Thoughtful Questions*: When meeting practitioners, show genuine curiosity. This creates meaningful conversations and could lead to future collaborations.
- *Support Practitioner-Led Businesses*: Purchasing herbal products or attending paid workshops is a great way to support small-scale herbalists while gaining access to their expertise.

These resources are just a starting point. Use them to enrich your understanding of herbal remedies and build a solid foundation of holistic knowledge. Whether you lean into the wisdom of books, join thriving online communities, or seek mentorship through practitioners, every step takes you closer to a deeper connection with nature's healing power.

Conclusion

Thank you for taking the time to explore this guide on Amish herbal remedies. By doing so, you've embarked on a meaningful path of rediscovery, grounded in tradition, nature, and intentional wellness. Your curiosity and willingness to learn are commendable, as they not only empower you to care for yourself but also deepen your connection to the natural world.

Amish herbal remedies serve as a gentle reminder that health doesn't have to be complicated. These time-honored practices tap into the earth's natural offerings, providing tools that nourish both your body and spirit. They reflect a philosophy of living simply, mindfully, and with respect for nature's balance. Whether it's brewing a comforting cup of tea, using a handcrafted salve, or growing herbs on your windowsill, each small step you take builds towards a healthier, more intentional life.

If there's one key takeaway from this guide, it's that wellness is a continuous, evolving process. You don't need to make drastic changes or master all the techniques at once. What matters most is starting where you are. Maybe that means trying your hand at a basic herbal tea blend or experimenting with making a tincture. These small but impactful actions offer an opportunity to engage with your health in a way that feels personal and manageable.

Stay curious as you expand your knowledge. Herbs have unique stories and benefits, and exploring them can be an enriching, lifelong experience. Seek out ways to learn more, whether that's joining workshops, engaging with like-minded communities, or even sharing what you've learned with family and friends. The more you surround yourself with resources and support, the more confident and inspired you'll feel in your herbal wellness practice.

Honor and trust your intuition as you go. Every body is different, and your experience with herbs will guide you toward what works best. Be patient with yourself and the remedies. They may take time to work, but this gradual, balanced approach is what makes herbalism so gentle yet effective. It's a process to savor, from cultivating a mindful routine to enjoying the benefits of natural, harmonious living.

Above all, give yourself credit for exploring an approach to health that values balance, prevention, and connection with nature. You're choosing to prioritize your well-being in a way that aligns with timeless principles of sustainability and care. This isn't just about remedies; it's about nurturing a lifestyle that fosters peace, gratitude, and respect for the earth.

Your herbal wellness journey doesn't end here. It's an ongoing practice of learning, experimenting, and integrating. By staying open-minded and intentional, you'll continue to discover new insights and deepen your connection to herbal healing.

FAQs

What are Amish herbal remedies?

Amish herbal remedies are traditional, plant-based practices used to promote wellness and prevent illness. These remedies rely on natural ingredients such as herbs, roots, and flowers, often prepared as teas, tinctures, poultices, or salves. They emphasize treating the root cause of ailments rather than just symptoms, reflecting a holistic approach to health.

Are Amish herbal remedies safe for everyone?

While most remedies are gentle and safe, some herbs can interact with medications or cause allergic reactions, especially for those with pre-existing health conditions or sensitivities. It's important to consult a healthcare provider if you're pregnant, nursing, taking medications, or have chronic illnesses before using herbal remedies.

How do I get started with Amish herbal remedies?

Start small by choosing one or two remedies that address your specific needs. For example, drink chamomile tea for relaxation or try a peppermint salve for muscle pain. You can also begin growing simple herbs like basil, mint, or lavender and experiment with preparing herbal teas or tinctures at home. Focus on learning basic techniques and adjust as you become more confident.

Where can I find high-quality herbs for these remedies?

You can source high-quality herbs by growing your own, purchasing from local farmers' markets, or ordering through reputable online suppliers. Always look for organic, pesticide-free options to ensure maximum potency and safety. Verify the source and avoid buying herbs from unknown or questionable vendors.

What are the most commonly used herbs in Amish remedies?

Some commonly used herbs include echinacea for immune support, chamomile for relaxation and digestion, peppermint for headaches and nausea, calendula for skin healing, and elderberry for colds and flu. Each herb has unique properties, making it versatile for various health applications.

How long does it take for herbal remedies to work?

Herbal remedies often work gradually and require consistent use. Timeframes vary depending on the remedy and individual factors. Immediate relief may be felt with remedies like peppermint tea for digestion, but long-term benefits, such as improved immunity with echinacea, might take weeks of regular use.

How can I incorporate Amish herbal remedies into my daily routine?

You can integrate remedies into your routine by pairing them with existing habits. For example, drink herbal tea in place of coffee, use a calming salve before bedtime, or add a tincture to your morning water. Creating small rituals around these remedies helps you build consistent habits and enhances mindfulness in your wellness practices.

References and Helpful Links

Strusnik, B. (2023, February 13). Amish health secrets. https://amishrules.com/amish-health-secrets/

samanthapriceshop. (n.d.). Amish Herbal and Natural Remedies (Hardcover). Samanthapriceshop. https://samanthapriceauthor.com/products/amish-herbal-and-natural-remedies-hardcover?srsltid=AfmBOorN2xMCSLbe2EVy_rIPd6mW2rqNCBqGUFBeUCa0jOXiMB4kYM6

Harris, M. (2024, October 27). 15 essentials the Amish always have on hand to survive anything — do you? - survival world. Survival World. https://www.survivalworld.com/preparedness/15-essentials-the-amish-always-have-on-hand-to-survive-anything-do-you/

Quillin, P. (n.d.). Amish Folk Medicine : Home remedies using foods, herbs and Vi. Quillin, Patrick: 9781886898004 - AbeBooks. https://www.abebooks.com/9781886898004/Amish-Folk-Medicine-Home-Remedies-1886898006/plp

Weber, C., Corneman, A., & Cin, A. D. (2021). Amish burn treatment meets a major trauma centre: success with cooperation. Plastic Surgery Case Studies, 7. https://doi.org/10.1177/2513826x211019577

Canning the Amish Way: Amish canning recipes plus home . . . (n.d.). Goodreads. https://www.goodreads.com/book/show/4424112-canning-the-amish-way

Chappell, S. (2019, December 18). A beginner's guide to making herbal salves and lotions. Healthline. https://www.healthline.com/health/diy-herbal-salves

www.ingramcontent.com/pod-product-compliance
Lightning Source LLC
LaVergne TN
LVHW012029060526
838201LV00061B/4525